The pain stethoscope:
A clinician's guide to measuring pain

The pain stethoscope: A clinician's guide to measuring pain

Mark P Jensen
Professor and Vice Chair for Research
Department of Rehabilitation Medicine
University of Washington School of Medicine
Seattle, WA, USA

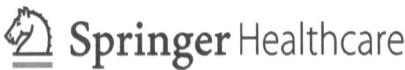

Published by Springer Healthcare Ltd, 236 Gray's Inn Road, London, WC1X 8HB, UK.

www.springerhealthcare.com

© 2011 Springer Healthcare, a part of Springer Science+Business Media.

British Library Cataloguing-in-Publication Data.

A catalogue record for this book is available from the British Library.

ISBN 978-1-907673-22-1

Although every effort has been made to ensure that drug doses and other information are presented accurately in this publication, the ultimate responsibility rests with the prescribing physician. Neither the publisher nor the authors can be held responsible for errors or for any consequences arising from the use of the information contained herein. Any product mentioned in this publication should be used in accordance with the prescribing information prepared by the manufacturers. No claims or endorsements are made for any drug or compound at present under clinical investigation.

Project editor: Tamsin Curtis
Designer: Joe Harvey
Artworker: Sissan Mollerfors
Production: Marina Maher

Contents

Author biography   vii
Acknowledgment   viii
Dedication   viii

1 **Introduction**   **1**
   Measuring pain in clinical practice   1
   How to use this book   2

2 **Measuring pain intensity**   **3**
   0–10 Numerical Rating Scale   4
   4-Point Verbal Rating Scale   5
   FACES Pain Scale – Revised   5

3 **Measuring pain quality**   **9**
   Pain Quality Assessment Scale – Revised edition   9
   Leeds Assessment of Neuropathic Symptoms and Signs   10

4 **Measuring pain location**   **17**
   Pain drawing   17

5 **Measuring pain behavior**   **19**
   PROMIS Pain Behavior Short Form   19

6 **Measuring pain interference**   **23**
   Pain Interference Subscale of the Brief Pain Inventory   23

7 **Measuring sleep quality**   **29**
   Medical Outcomes Study Sleep Problem Index   29

8 **Measuring depression**   **33**
   Patient Health Questionnaire-2   33

9 Measuring general physical functioning   **37**

PROMIS Physical Function Short Forms   37

10 Measuring alcohol and drug use   **43**

Two-item conjoint screen   43

Behavioral Risk Factor Surveillance System assessing alcohol use   43

11 Measuring global improvement and satisfaction with pain care   **47**

Five-point patient rating of satisfaction with pain management   47

Patient Global Impression of Change   48

12 References   **51**

Author biography

Mark P. Jensen, PhD, is Professor and Vice Chair for Research in the Department of Rehabilitation Medicine, University of Washington School of Medicine, where he has been on faculty since 1990. Dr Jensen's research program focuses on the development and evaluation of measures of pain, pain beliefs, and pain coping strategies, as well as on the development and evaluation of psychosocial pain interventions. He is the author or co-author of over 250 scientific articles and book chapters.

Acknowledgment

This book benefited greatly from the advice of my wife and partner, Lisa C. Murphy, M.D., whose clinical experience helped me to determine the measures and information that should be included. She also provided valuable editorial help. The book would not have been as useful or clear without her help.

Dedication

This book is dedicated to the many organizations that work to ease the suffering associated with chronic pain, including: The American Chronic Pain Association, The American Pain Society, and The International Association for the Study of Pain.

Chapter 1

Introduction

Measuring pain in clinical practice

After the common cold, pain is the most common reason for health care visits. Although estimates of the prevalence of chronic pain range from 8% to 60% or more, depending on how chronic pain is defined and the populations studied [1], there is a consensus that chronic pain has profound personal costs to individuals, and economic costs to society. One study has estimated that pain results in an annual cost of $61.2 billion per year in the United States in terms of loss of productive work time alone [2]. Taking into account the additional dollars spent on health care, compensation, and litigation, the total cost of pain in the United States is likely to exceed $100 billion annually [3].

In order to treat pain effectively, clinicians need to be able to assess pain and its effects on functioning. However, hundreds, if not thousands, of different measures of pain and pain-related domains exist. Surprisingly, despite the fact that much is known about the strengths and weaknesses of existing measures [4,5], there does not yet exist a simple and brief guide that describes the most useful and psychometrically sound pain measures for healthcare providers.

This book briefly describes the most reliable and valid measures of ten key domains that clinicians treating patients with pain should consider assessing. These domains include:
- pain intensity;
- pain quality;
- pain location;
- pain behavior;
- pain interference;

- sleep quality;
- depression;
- general physical functioning;
- alcohol and drug use history; and
- global improvement and satisfaction with pain care.

The measures included in book were selected based on the availability of evidence supporting their reliability and validity, as well as their practical utility in the clinical setting. Also, all of the measures published in this book can be copied for use within the clinical practice, although some of the measures do require permission for use in clinical trials.

Assessment of each key domain is covered in a single chapter (Chapters 1–10), and each chapter provides:

- a brief description of the domain to be assessed and its clinical relevance;
- a copy of the measure(s) recommended to assess the domain, in a form that makes administration easy;
- administration instructions; and
- interpretation information.

How to use this book

In order to make the book portable and easy to use in a clinical setting, detailed information about the strengths and weaknesses of the measures presented relative to other existing measures is not included. Instead, the chapters present only information that is most useful for the practicing clinician, including information about critical cut-offs when they are known (e.g., for determining if a patient likely meets criteria for depression, or for having neuropathic versus non-neuropathic pain) and meaningful differences (e.g., for determining how much change in a measure's score is needed in order to determine that meaningful change has occurred). Sources for more in-depth information about each measure are cited, however, for those readers who desire this information. The book has been purposefully published at a size that is both easy to carry in a pocket and can be photocopied (at a 170% increase) onto an 8½" X 11" piece of paper if the clinician wants hard copy versions of the measures to administer.

Chapter 2

Measuring pain intensity

Pain intensity is the magnitude or severity of perceived pain. It is the pain domain most often measured in the clinical setting because it is usually the primary target of pain treatment. Although it is possible to ask patients to rate their *current* pain intensity, clinicians (and patients) are usually more interested in treating the patient's "usual" or average pain. However, when patients are asked to estimate their average pain intensity over a specified period of time (say, the last week), different patients use different strategies for computing an average score [6]. For example, some might attempt to take into account the entire time period – including those times when they might have experienced no pain – when computing an average. Others might compute an average by taking into account only those times when they felt pain. Thus, two patients with the same experience might provide two different 'average' pain scores. This means that one person's average pain score is not easily comparable to another's. Also, when patients are asked to rate their average pain in the past week, there is a tendency for them to over-estimate this pain by about 10%, relative to an average score made up of multiple ratings of current pain obtained over that same week. This tendency to over-estimate past pain has not been observed for recall ratings of average pain in the past day, however.

Despite the problems with asking patients to rate their average pain, scores from simple pain rating scales remain amazingly robust with respect to their ability to detect clinically meaningful changes in pain over time. The three ratings scales that are most practical for assessing pain intensity in clinical settings are the 0–10 Numerical Rating Scale

(NRS), the 4-Point Verbal Rating Scale (VRS), and the 6-point FACES Pain Scale – Revised (FPS-R).

0–10 Numerical Rating Scale

The pain intensity rating scale that has been determined by experts to have the most strengths and fewest weaknesses is the 0–10 NRS (Figure 2.1). Patients can be asked to use this scale to rate their current pain or their least, average, or most/worst pain over a specific time period. To administer the 0–10 NRS, the clinician asks the patient: *"Please tell me (or circle if using a print-off copy) the number that best represents your average [or current, least, or worst] pain intensity over the past seven days [or 24 hours] on a 0 to 10 scale, where 0 = 'No pain' and 10 = 'Pain as intense as you can imagine.'"* Patients will occasionally elect to provide a number between two integers (e.g., *"7 to 8"* or *"about 7 and a half"*), which can be allowed, as some people are able to detect 20 or more different distinct levels of pain intensity.

The number that the patient selects is his or her NRS score. Research shows that these scores can be used to classify a patient's pain as mild, moderate, or severe [7]. Mild pain intensity (a score of 1–4 on the 0–10 NRS) is pain that is noticeable, but usually has relative little effect on day-to-day functioning. Moderate pain (a score of 5–6) is pain that is starting to interfere with some areas of functioning, such as socializing, sleep, and mood, but does not produce marked interference across a broad range of activities. Severe pain intensity (a score of 7–10) is pain that has become a central aspect of the patient's life, and that produces significant interference across a wide range of activities.

Treatment rarely eliminates chronic pain completely, so the goal of treatment is usually to reduce pain intensity as much as possible, while limiting the chances of negative treatment side effects. Although any reduction in pain intensity can be viewed as a positive thing – especially if the treatment producing this reduction has little cost and very few negative side effects – research supports decreases of approximately 30% (or 2 points on the 0–10 scale) as clinically meaningful to most patients [8]. Perhaps not coincidentally, a pain decrease of 30% often reflects a shift in pain intensity classification; from severe (7–10) to moderate (5–6), or moderate to mild (1–4).

4-Point Verbal Rating Scale

The 4-Point VRS (Figure 2.2) consists of a list of four pain intensity descriptors: no pain, mild pain, moderate pain, and severe pain. As with the 0–10 NRS, patients can use the 4-Point VRS to rate their current pain or their recollection of least, worst, and average pain over a specified period of time. Patients are asked to indicate the word or phrase that best describes their pain intensity (e.g., *"Please look at this list of words and tell me which one best describes the average pain intensity you have experienced in the past week"*). Responses are then coded from 0 to 3, with 0 = "No pain," 1 = "Mild pain," 2 = "Moderate pain," and 3 = "Severe pain."

The 4-Point VRS cannot be used to detect small changes in pain intensity, and is therefore less sensitive than the 0–10 NRS to changes in pain. For this reason, most clinicians will elect to use the 0–10 NRS instead of the 4-Point VRS. However, there is the occasional patient who is not able to use a numerical rating scale, and these patients may require a more simple categorical scale such as the 4-Point VRS. Even if the 4-Point VRS is not sensitive to very small changes in pain intensity, however, it is certainly sensitive to larger and perhaps more clinically meaningful changes. A reasonable treatment goal would be to reduce pain from one VRS response to another (e.g., severe to moderate), with an endpoint goal of "mild pain" if "no pain" is not possible given the patient's pain condition.

FACES Pain Scale – Revised

The FPS-R (Figure 2.3) consists of six drawings of faces that reflect different expressions that might be expected giving increasing levels of pain intensity [9]. Patients are shown the six faces (but not the numbers associated with each face) and told, *"These faces show how much something can hurt. This face* [point to left-most face] *shows **no pain**. The faces show more and more pain* [point to each from left to right] *up to this one* [point to right-most face], *which shows **a great deal of pain**. Point to* *the face that shows how much you hurt [right now/in the past week].*" The patient's FPS-R score is the number associated with each face.

The FPS-R was initially designed to be used for young children (as young as 4 years old) who might have difficulty understanding the 0–10 NRS or the words on the 4-Point VRS. It could also potentially be used with individuals who might have difficulties communicating in English.

0–10 Numerical Rating Scale

1	2	3	4	5	6	7	8	9	10
No pain									Pain as intense as you can imagine

Figure 2.1 The 0–10 Numerical Rating Scale.

0–3 Verbal Rating Scale

☐ No pain

☐ Mild pain

☐ Moderate pain

☐ Severe pain

Figure 2.2 The 0–3 Verbal Rating Scale.

6-Point FACES Pain Scale – Revised

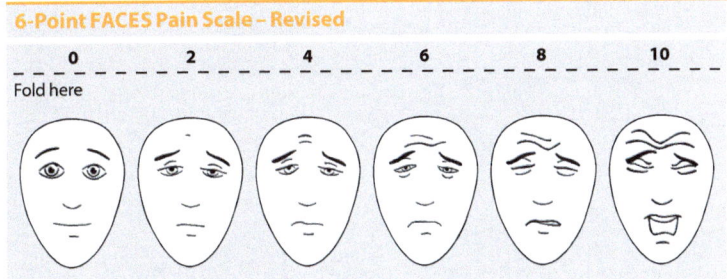

Figure 2.3 FACES Pain Scale – Revised. The FACES Pain Scale – Revised is available for clinical use on www.usask.ca/childpain/fpsr. It is free-of-charge and intended for clinicians to use as a resource. ©2001 International Association for the Study of Pain (IASP). Reproduced with permission from the IASP [9].

Chapter 3

Measuring pain quality

The experience of pain includes much more than its intensity and location. It can also have many different qualities, such as "hot" or "electrical" or "aching." Measures of these pain qualities have been developed for two primary purposes:

- to describe the pain qualities a patient experiences and detect changes in these qualities with treatment; and
- to help diagnose the pain problem as being due to nerve damage (neuropathic pain) or due to the stimulation of undamaged nociceptors (nociceptive pain).

Determining the type of pain (neuropathic vs nociceptive) experienced by the patient has important clinical implications, since treatments that benefit each pain type differ [10,11].

A useful measure for the first purpose is the Pain Quality Assessment Scale – Revised edition (PQAS-R) [12]. One of the best measures for determining if a pain problem is primarily neuropathic or nociceptive is the Leeds Assessment of Neuropathic Symptoms and Signs (LANSS).

Pain Quality Assessment Scale – Revised edition

The PQAS-R includes 20 questions that assess all of the most common pain qualities associated with clinical pain conditions (Figure 3.1). Patients are asked to rate the severity of each pain quality on a 0–10 numerical rating scale. The primary reason to assess multiple pain qualities in addition to global pain intensity is that treatments might have little measureable effects on overall pain intensity, but may result in significant relief in certain pain qualities. These important effects would go unnoticed if only pain intensity were assessed. Although research has not yet deter-mined how much change in a pain quality might be needed in order for that change to be deemed meaningful, it would be reasonable to use the same standards for pain quality severity as those used for pain intensity; that is, a reduction of 30% (or about 2 points on a 0–10 scale) could be deemed clinically meaningful.

Leeds Assessment of Neuropathic Symptoms and Signs

The LANSS pain scale was designed to distinguish neuropathic from nociceptive pain (Figure 5) [13]. The LANSS is administered by a clini-cian and requires the patient to report on the degree of dysesthesia (e.g., "tingling" or "pins and needles"), thermal quality (e.g., "hot" or "burning"), paroxysmal pain (e.g., "electric" or "jumping"), autonomic dysfunction (e.g., "mottled" or "pink" skin), and allodynia (e.g., "sensitive"). The items also include two sensory clinical tests:

1. for allodynia (abnormal pain evoked by gentle stroking with cotton wool); and
2. for hyperalgesia (pain evoked by a pin-prick).

The LANSS has shown a very high rate (85%) of accuracy in classifying patients has having neuropathic versus non-neuropathic pain in the origi-nal development sample, which was largely replicated in a cross-validation sample (82% accuracy) [13]. This high rate of accuracy has also been replicated in additional samples of patients with chronic pain [14,15].

To score the LANSS, simply sum the values in parentheses for both the five pain questionnaire items and the two sensory items. The LANSS score thus ranges from 0 to 24. Scores of less than 12 indicate that neuro-pathic mechanisms are unlikely to be contributing to the patient's pain, and scores ≥12 indicate that neuropathic mechanisms are likely to be contributing to the patient's pain problem.

Pain Quality Assessment Scale – Revised

Instructions: There are different aspects and types of pain that patients experience and that we are interested in measuring. Pain can feel sharp, hot, and achy. Some pains may feel like they are very superficial (at skin-level), or they may feel like they are from deep inside your body. Some people can feel these different types of pain at the same time.

The Pain Quality Assessment Scale helps us measure these and other different aspects of your pain. For one patient, a pain might feel extremely hot and burning, but not at all achy, while another patient may not experience any burning pain, but feel like their pain is very achy. Therefore, we expect that you may rate higher on some of the scales and lower on others.

We are asking you to rate the intensity or severity of the different types of pain you have felt over the past week **on average**, using a question like the one below. We realize that it can be difficult to make these estimates for some of the items, but please give us your best estimate.

Place an "X" through the number that best describes your pain. For example:

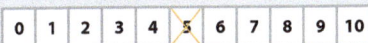

And remember, we want you to rate how severe each pain type has been **on average** during the past week.

1. Please use the scale below to tell us how **intense** your pain is.

2. Please use the scale below to tell us how **sharp** your pain feels. Words used to describe "sharp" feelings include "like a knife", "like a spike", "jabbing", or "like jolts."

3. Please use the scale below to tell us how **hot** your pain feels. Words used to describe very hot pain include "burning" and "on fire."

4. Please use the scale below to tell us how **dull** your pain feels. Words used to describe very dull pain include "like a dull toothache", "dull pain", and "like a bruise."

5. Please use the scale below to tell us how **cold** your pain feels. Words used to describe very cold pain include "like ice" and "freezing."

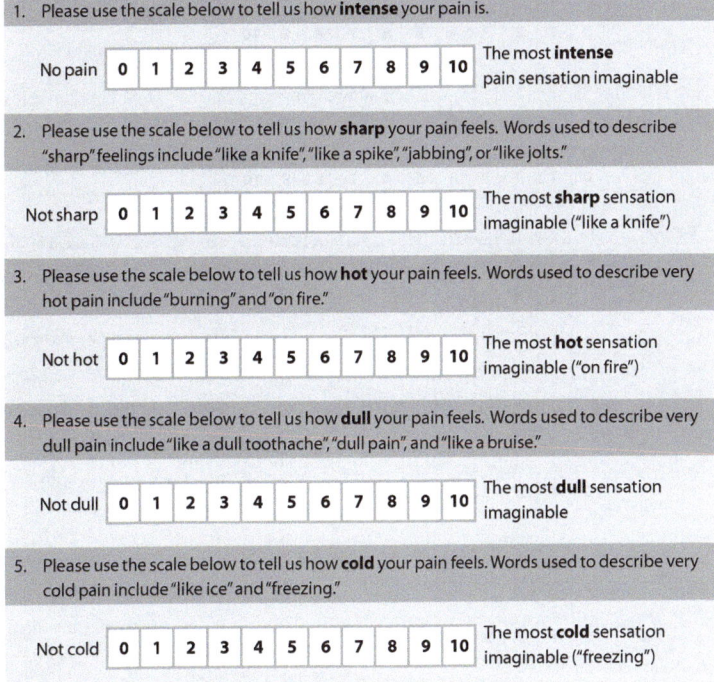

Figure 3.1 Pain Quality Assessment Scale – Revised (continues overleaf).

Pain Quality Assessment Scale – Revised (continued)

6. Please use the scale below to tell us how **sensitive** your skin is to light touch or clothing. Words used to describe sensitive skin include "like sunburned skin", and "raw skin."

    Not sensitive | 0 1 2 3 4 5 6 7 8 9 10 | The most **sensitive** sensation imaginable ("raw skin")

7. Please use the scale below to tell us how **tender** your pain is when something has pressed against it over the past week. Another word used to describe tender pain is "like a bruise."

    Not tender | 0 1 2 3 4 5 6 7 8 9 10 | The most **tender** sensation imaginable ("like a bruise")

8. Please use the scale below to tell us how **itchy** your pain feels. Words used to describe itchy pain include "like poison oak" and "like a mosquito bite."

    Not itchy | 0 1 2 3 4 5 6 7 8 9 10 | The most **itchy** sensation imaginable ("like poison oak")

9. Please use the scale below to tell us how much your pain has felt like it has been **shooting** over the past week. Another word used to describe shooting pain is "zapping."

    Not shooting | 0 1 2 3 4 5 6 7 8 9 10 | The most **shooting** sensation imaginable ("zapping")

10. Please use the scale below to tell us how **numb** your pain has felt over the past week. A phrase that can be used to describe numb pain is "like it is asleep".

    Not numb | 0 1 2 3 4 5 6 7 8 9 10 | The most **numb** sensation imaginable ("asleep")

11. Please use the scale below to tell us how much your pain sensations have felt **electrical** over the past week. Words used to describe electrical pain include "shocks," "lightning," and "sparking."

    Not electrical | 0 1 2 3 4 5 6 7 8 9 10 | The most **electrical** sensation imaginable ("shocks")

12. Please use the scale below to tell us how **tingling** your pain has felt over the past week. Words used to describe tingling pain include "like pins and needles" and "prickling."

    Not tingling | 0 1 2 3 4 5 6 7 8 9 10 | The most **tingling** sensation imaginable ("pins and needles")

13. Please use the scale below to tell us how **cramping** your pain has felt over the past week. Words used to describe cramping pain include "squeezing" and "tight."

    Not cramping | 0 1 2 3 4 5 6 7 8 9 10 | The most **cramping** sensation imaginable ("squeezing")

Figure 3.1 Pain Quality Assessment Scale – Revised (continues opposite).

Pain Quality Assessment Scale – Revised (continued)

14. Please use the scale below to tell us how **radiating** your pain has felt over the past week. Another word used to describe radiating pain is "spreading."

Not radiating | 0 1 2 3 4 5 6 7 8 9 10 | The most **radiating** sensation imaginable ("spreading")

15. Please use the scale below to tell us how **throbbing** your pain has felt over the past week. Another word used to describe throbbing pain is "pounding."

Not throbbing | 0 1 2 3 4 5 6 7 8 9 10 | The most **throbbing** sensation imaginable ("pounding")

16. Please use the scale below to tell us how **aching** your pain has felt over the past week. Another word used to describe aching pain is "like a toothache."

Not aching | 0 1 2 3 4 5 6 7 8 9 10 | The most **aching** sensation imaginable ("like a toothache")

17. How **heavy** has your pain felt over the past week? (e.g., "pressure" and "weighted down").

Not heavy | 0 1 2 3 4 5 6 7 8 9 10 | The most **heavy** sensation imaginable

18. Now that you have told us the different types of pain sensations you have felt, we want you to tell us overall how **unpleasant** your pain has been to you over the past week. Words used to describe very unpleasant pain include "annoying," "bothersome," "miserable," and "intolerable." Remember, pain can have a low intensity but still feel extremely **unpleasant**, and some kinds of pain can have a high intensity but be very tolerable. With this scale, please tell us how unpleasant your pain feels.

Not unpleasant | 0 1 2 3 4 5 6 7 8 9 10 | The most **unpleasant** sensation imaginable ("intolerable")

19. Finally, we want you to give us an estimate of the severity of your deep versus surface pain over the past week. We want you to rate each location of pain separately. We realize that it can be difficult to make these estimates, and most likely it will be a best guess, but please give us your best estimate.

How intense is your **deep** pain?

No **deep** pain | 0 1 2 3 4 5 6 7 8 9 10 | The most **intense deep** pain sensation imaginable

How intense is your **surface** pain?

No **surface** pain | 0 1 2 3 4 5 6 7 8 9 10 | The most **intense surface** pain sensation imaginable

Figure 3.1 Pain Quality Assessment Scale – Revised (continues overleaf).

Pain Quality Assessment Scale – Revised (PQAS-R) (continued)

20. Pain can also have different time qualities. For some people, the pain comes and goes and so they have some moments that are completely without pain; in other words the pain "comes and goes." This is called **intermittent** pain. Others are never pain free, but their pain types and pain severity can vary from one moment to the next. This is called **variable** pain. For these people, the increases can be severe, so that they feel they have moments of very intense pain ("breakthrough" pain), but at other times they can feel lower levels of pain ("background" pain). Still, they are never pain free. Other people have pain that really does not change that much from one moment to another. This is called **stable** pain. Which of these best describes the time pattern of your pain (please select only one):

☐ I have **intermittent** pain (I feel pain sometimes but I am pain-free at other times)

☐ I have **variable** pain ("background" pain all the time, but also moments of more pain, or even severe "breakthrough" pain or varying types of pain)

☐ I have **stable** pain (constant pain that does not change very much from one moment to another, and no pain-free periods)

Figure 3.1 Pain Quality Assessment Scale – Revised (PQAS-R) (continued). Clinicians can use the PQAS-R at no cost for clinical care, and investigators can use the PQAS-R at no cost in non-funded clinical studies. Instructions for obtaining permission to use the PQAS-R in research are available on the MAPI Research Trust website (www.mapi-trust.org). ©2010 Galer, Gammaitoni, and Jensen. All rights reserved, reproduced with permission from Jensen et al. [12].

The Leeds Assessment of Neuropathic Symptoms and Signs

Name: Date:

This pain scale can help to determine whether the nerves that are carrying your pain signals are working normally or not. It is important to find this out in case different treatments are needed to control your pain.

A. Pain questionnaire

Think about how your pain has felt over the last week. Please say whether any of the descriptions match your pain exactly.

1. **Does your pain feel like strange, unpleasant sensations in your skin? Words like pricking, tingling, pins and needles might describe these sensations**

a. NO – My pain doesn't really feel like this (0)

b. YES – I get these sensations quite a lot (5)

2. **Does your pain make the skin in the painful area look different from normal? Words like mottled or looking more red or pink might describe the appearance**

a. NO – My pain doesn't affect the color of my skin (0)

b. YES – I've noticed that the pain does make my skin look different from normal (5)

3. **Does your pain make the affected skin abnormally sensitive to touch? Getting unpleasant sensations when lightly stroking the skin, or getting pain when wearing tight clothes might describe the abnormal sensitivity**

a. NO – My pain doesn't make my skin abnormally sensitive in that area (0)

b. YES – My skin seems abnormally sensitive to touch in that area (3)

Figure 3.2 The Leeds Assessment of Neuropathic Symptoms and Signs (continues overleaf).

The Leeds Assessment of Neuropathic Symptoms and Signs (continued)

4. Does your pain come on suddenly and in bursts for no apparent reason when you're still. Words like electric shocks, jumping and bursting describe these sensations

a. NO – My pain doesn't really feel like this (0)

b. YES – I get these sensations quite a lot (2)

5. Does your pain feel as if the skin temperature in the painful area has changed abnormally? Words like hot and burning describe these sensations

a. NO – I don't really get these sensations (0)

b. YES – I get these sensations quite a lot (1)

B. Sensory testing

Skin sensitivity can be examined by comparing the painful area with a contralateral or adjacent non-painful area for the presence of allodynia and an altered pin-prick threshold (PPT).

1. Allodynia

Examine the response to lightly stroking cotton wool across the non-painful area and then the painful area. If normal sensations are experienced in the non-painful site, but pain or unpleasant sensations (tingling, nausea) are experienced in the painful area when stroking, allodynia is present.

a. NO – normal sensation in both areas (0)

b. YES – allodynia in painful area only (5)

2. Altered pin-prick threshold

Determine the pin-prick threshold by comparing the response to a 23 gauge (blue) needle mounted inside a 2-mL syringe barrel placed gently on to the skin in a non-painful and then painful areas.

If a sharp pin-prick is felt in the non-painful area, but a different sensation is experienced in the painful area e.g., none / blunt only (raised PPT) or a very painful sensation (lowered PPT), an altered PPT is present.

If a pin-prick is not felt in either area, mount the syringe onto the needle to increase the weight and repeat.

a. NO – equal sensation in both areas (0)

b. YES – altered PPT in painful area (3)

Figure 3.2 The Leeds Assessment of Neuropathic Symptoms and Signs (continued).
Reproduced with permission from the International Association for the Study of Pain [8].

Chapter 4

Measuring pain location

Knowledge about pain location has important clinical implications. It is helpful for making a diagnosis (e.g., arthritis pain tends to be in the joints, "widespread" pain conditions such as fibromyalgia tend to be at many locations). Moreover, the effects of pain on a patient's life varies as a function of pain locations; pain in the lower back and hands or arms has a larger negative impact on functioning than pain at other locations, and pain that covers more areas of the body – also known as "pain extent" – has a larger negative impact on functioning than pain that is more focal.

The most common method clinicians use to assess pain location is to simply ask the patient, *"Tell me where you hurt?"* The location(s) of pain stated by the patient can then be documented in the medical record. However, this method does not allow for an ongoing record of pain extent (the percentage of body area in pain). The pain drawing was therefore developed to help record pain extent.

Pain drawing

The pain drawing consists of a line drawing of the front and back of a body (Figure 4.1) [16]. Patients are asked to indicate the location of their pain on the drawing by shading in all of the body areas that are in pain. Scoring the pain drawing is simple; to identify the specific location(s), one need only observe the areas of the body that have been shaded. The pain extent score is computed by summing the number of areas on the drawing that have been at least partially shaded. Thus, the pain extent score can range from 0 to 45.

Pain drawing

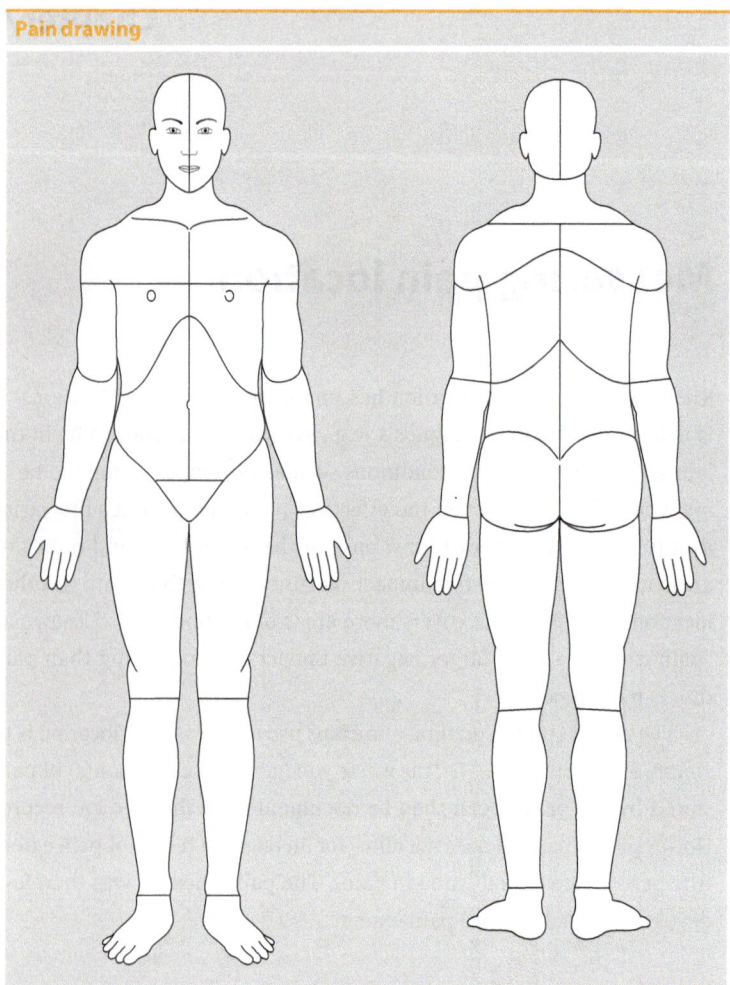

Figure 4.1 Pain drawing. Reproduced with permission from the International Association for the Study of Pain [11].

Chapter 5

Measuring pain behavior

Pain behaviors are the things that patients do when they experience pain. They can include efforts to cope with or manage the pain, such as limping, body posturing, and resting. They also include behaviors that communicate pain to others, such as verbal complaints of pain, groans, and facial expressions. If it can be observed and counted, and if it is associated with pain, it is a pain behavior.

The presence of a significant amount of pain behavior is an objective indication that the patient is at risk for developing more problems over time. This is due, in part, to the fact that pain behaviors may elicit solicitous responses from those in the patient's immediate environment (e.g., a spouse, relative, or friend), who can reinforce that behavior, and therefore contribute to higher reports of pain and dysfunction over time. Also, some pain behaviors – excessive resting or unusual posturing, for example – can contribute to muscle atrophy and weakness, which can then also contribute to greater pain and dysfunction. High levels of pain behavior suggest that treatment, often in the form of active physical therapy, is indicated. One of the most recent pain behavior measures that has been developed is the Patient-Reported Outcomes Measurement Information System (PROMIS) Pain Behavior item bank [17].

PROMIS Pain Behavior Short Form

Seven items from the PROMIS Pain Behavior item bank make up the PROMIS Pain Behavior Short Form (Figure 5.1). Patients rate the frequency that they displayed each pain behavior listed (when they felt pain) in the past week on a 6-point scale from "Had no pain" or "Never" to "Always."

Each response has a score associated with it from 1 through 6 (i.e., "Had no pain" = 1; "Never" = 2; "Rarely" = 3; "Sometimes" = 4; "Often" = 5; "Always" = 6), and the patient's raw pain behavior score is the sum of all items; thus, scores can range from 7 to 42. One of the strengths of all of the PROMIS measures, including the PROMIS Pain Behavior Short Form scale, is that raw scores can be transformed into T-scores. A T-score is a standardized metric with a mean of 50 and a standard deviation of 10, based on a normative sample. Because the PROMIS measures were developed using a normative sample that represented in the United States general population, a patient who has a T-score of 60 would be reporting a level of pain behaviors that is substantially (one standard deviation unit) higher than in the United States normative sample. Table 1 can be used to convert a patient's raw Pain Behavior score into a T-score.

Research identifying specific cut-offs that represent problematic levels of pain behaviors and treatment goals has not yet been performed. However, a decrease of at least one-half of a standard deviation (T-score decrease of 5 points) would likely indicate a meaningful decrease [18]. A final endpoint goal raw score of 14 (T-score of 50.1, relative to the normative sample, indicating no pain behaviors on average) is probably not realistic for most patients with chronic pain. A final raw score of 21 (T-score of 56.4) would indicate that the patient is reporting that he or she only rarely engages in the seven pain behaviors on the PROMIS Pain Behavior Short Form scale, on average (Table 5.1). Such a score would likely be indicative of the patient doing well in this outcome domain, and would be a reasonable endpoint treatment goal.

PROMIS Pain Behavior Short Form

Please respond to each item by marking one box per row

In the past 7 days…

1. When I was in pain I became irritable

☐ Had no pain   ☐ Never   ☐ Rarely   ☐ Sometimes   ☐ Often   ☐ Always

2. When I was in pain I grimaced

☐ Had no pain   ☐ Never   ☐ Rarely   ☐ Sometimes   ☐ Often   ☐ Always

3. When I was in pain I moved extremely slowly

☐ Had no pain   ☐ Never   ☐ Rarely   ☐ Sometimes   ☐ Often   ☐ Always

4. When I was in pain I moved stiffly

☐ Had no pain   ☐ Never   ☐ Rarely   ☐ Sometimes   ☐ Often   ☐ Always

5. When I was in pain I called out for someone to help me

☐ Had no pain   ☐ Never   ☐ Rarely   ☐ Sometimes   ☐ Often   ☐ Always

6. When I was in pain I isolated myself from others

☐ Had no pain   ☐ Never   ☐ Rarely   ☐ Sometimes   ☐ Often   ☐ Always

7. When I was in pain I thrashed

☐ Had no pain   ☐ Never   ☐ Rarely   ☐ Sometimes   ☐ Often   ☐ Always

Figure 5.1 PROMIS Pain Behavior Short Form. ©2009 PROMIS Health Organization and PROMIS Cooperative Group. Reproduced with permission from PROMIS [19].

PROMIS Pain Behavior Short Form conversion table

Raw score	T-score	SE	Raw score	T-score	SE
7	36.7	5.1	25	59.2	1.5
8	42.5	2.3	26	59.9	1.4
9	44.4	1.8	27	60.6	1.4
10	45.7	1.6	28	61.2	1.4
11	46.9	1.6	29	61.9	1.4
12	48.0	1.6	30	62.5	1.4
13	49.0	1.6	31	63.1	1.4
14	50.1	1.6	32	63.8	1.4
15	51.1	1.7	33	64.4	1.4
16	52.1	1.7	34	65.1	1.4
17	53.0	1.7	35	65.8	1.5
18	53.9	1.6	36	66.6	1.5
19	54.8	1.6	37	67.4	1.6
20	55.6	1.6	38	68.3	1.7
21	56.4	1.5	39	69.3	1.8
22	57.1	1.5	40	70.5	2.0
23	57.8	1.5	41	72.1	2.2
24	58.6	1.5	42	75.9	3.7

Table 5.1 PROMIS Pain Behavior Short Form conversion table. SE, standard error on T-score metric. ©2009 PROMIS Health Organization and PROMIS Cooperative Group. Reproduced with permission from PROMIS [19].

Chapter 6

Measuring pain interference

Chronic pain often has significant negative effects on a patient's overall quality of life, and effective pain treatments can and should result in a decrease in these negative effects. Clinicians can measure a number of quality of life domains that can be negatively influenced by pain such as sleep quality, depression, and general physical functioning (see Chapters 7, 8, and 9, respectively). However, as important as it is to monitor these quality of life domains, many factors in addition to pain intensity can influence them. For example, a patient may have difficulty sleeping because of anxiety or depression in additional to pain. When the clinician wants to assess the specific effects of *pain* on quality of life, it is best to use a measure of *pain interference*. The Pain Interference Subscale of the Brief Pain Inventory (BPI) is among the most commonly used measures of this construct [20].

Pain Interference Subscale of the Brief Pain Inventory

The original Pain Interference Subscale and a modified version of the Pain Interference Subscale from the BPI are presented in Figures 6.1a and 6.2b, respectively. The original BPI Pain Interference Subscale asks patients to indicate the extent to which pain interferes with seven quality of life domains (general activity, mood, walking ability, normal work [including housework], relations with other people, sleep, and enjoyment of life) on 0 ("Does not interfere") to 10 ("Completely interferes") numerical rating scales. The time period covered for the ratings can vary, depending on the goals of the assessment (e.g., the past 24 hours, the past week), although a 7-day period would be a reasonable time frame to use in many clinical settings.

The original BPI Pain Interference Subscale was modified to make it more useful for individuals with physical disabilities, many of whom have mobility limitations unrelated to pain that therefore makes the "Walking ability" item inappropriate [21–23]. These modifications included re-wording "Walking ability" to read "Mobility (ability to get around)" so that individuals in wheelchairs or who are otherwise unable to walk independently could respond to the item. The modifications also included the addition of five items so that the scale would reflect the key activity and participation domains identified in the International Classification of Functioning, Disability, and Health [24]. Specifically, items were added to assess the extent to which pain interferes with self-care, recreational activity, social activities, communication with others, and learning new information or skills. Evidence supports the reliability and validity of both the original and modified BPI Pain Interference sub-scales [21–23,25], including the ability of this measure to detect changes in pain with pain treatment [26–28].

Empirically derived BPI Pain Interference Subscale cut-off scores have not yet been established. However, until such cut offs are identified, it would be reasonable to anticipate that patients would respond to the 0–10 NRS of pain interference in ways that are similar to the way that they respond to 0–10 scales of pain intensity; that is, 0–4 may represent a "mild" level of interference, 5–6 a "moderate" level of interference, and 7–10 a "severe" level of interference. Similarly, as with the 0–10 scale of pain intensity, a decrease of 2 points or more would likely be viewed as meaningful to most patients.

Pain Interference Subscale of the Brief Pain Inventory

Instructions: Circle the one number that describes how, during the past week, pain has interfered with your...

A. General activity

Does not interfere | 0 1 2 3 4 5 6 7 8 9 10 | Completely interferes

B. Mood

Does not interfere | 0 1 2 3 4 5 6 7 8 9 10 | Completely interferes

C. Walking ability

Does not interfere | 0 1 2 3 4 5 6 7 8 9 10 | Completely interferes

D. Normal work (includes both work outside the home and housework)

Does not interfere | 0 1 2 3 4 5 6 7 8 9 10 | Completely interferes

E. Relations with other people

Does not interfere | 0 1 2 3 4 5 6 7 8 9 10 | Completely interferes

F. Sleep

Does not interfere | 0 1 2 3 4 5 6 7 8 9 10 | Completely interferes

G. Enjoyment of life

Does not interfere | 0 1 2 3 4 5 6 7 8 9 10 | Completely interferes

Figure 6.1a Pain Interference Subscale of the Brief Pain Inventory. There is no cost for using this scale in clinical settings, but permission is required for use in clinical trials and for commercial purposes. ©1991 Dr Charles S. Cleeland. Reproduced with permission from Cleeland [21].

Modified Pain Interference Subscale of the Brief Pain Inventory

Instructions: Circle the one number that describes how, during the past week, pain has interfered with your...

A. General activity

Does not interfere | 0 1 2 3 4 5 6 7 8 9 10 | Completely interferes

B. Mood

Does not interfere | 0 1 2 3 4 5 6 7 8 9 10 | Completely interferes

C. Mobility (ability to get around)

Does not interfere | 0 1 2 3 4 5 6 7 8 9 10 | Completely interferes

D. Normal work (includes both work outside the home and housework)

Does not interfere | 0 1 2 3 4 5 6 7 8 9 10 | Completely interferes

E. Relations with other people

Does not interfere | 0 1 2 3 4 5 6 7 8 9 10 | Completely interferes

F. Sleep

Does not interfere | 0 1 2 3 4 5 6 7 8 9 10 | Completely interferes

G. Enjoyment of life

Does not interfere | 0 1 2 3 4 5 6 7 8 9 10 | Completely interferes

H. Self-care

Does not interfere | 0 1 2 3 4 5 6 7 8 9 10 | Completely interferes

I. Recreational activities

Does not interfere | 0 1 2 3 4 5 6 7 8 9 10 | Completely interferes

Figure 6.2b Modified Pain Interference Subscale of the Brief Pain Inventory (continues opposite).

Modified Pain Interference Subscale of the Brief Pain Inventory (continued)

J. Social activities

Does not interfere	0	1	2	3	4	5	6	7	8	9	10	Completely interferes

K. Communication with others

Does not interfere	0	1	2	3	4	5	6	7	8	9	10	Completely interferes

L. Learning new information or skills

Does not interfere	0	1	2	3	4	5	6	7	8	9	10	Completely interferes

Figure 6.2b Modified Pain Interference Subscale of the Brief Pain Inventory (continued).
There is no cost for using this scale in clinical settings, but permission is required for use in clinical trials and for commercial purposes. ©1991 Dr Charles S. Cleeland. Reproduced with permission from Cleeland [20].

Chapter 7

Measuring sleep quality

Sleep problems are very common in patients with chronic pain. Studies indicate that 50–80% of patients with chronic pain report significant sleep difficulties [29–31], and sleep problems are more severe among those with chronic pain relative to those without chronic pain [32]. There is also preliminary evidence that sleep problems may contribute to increased pain [33], and that effective sleep treatment results in decreased pain [34,35]. It is therefore important that sleep problems be assessed in persons with chronic pain, and treated if indicated. The Medical Outcomes Study Sleep Problem Index is a validated measure of sleep quality that is also very easy to administer.

Medical Outcomes Study Sleep Problem Index

The nine items of the Medical Outcomes Study Sleep Problem Index II (SPI II) are part of the 12-item Medical Outcomes Study Sleep Scale [36], and are shown in Figure 7.1. Scoring the SPI II results in a final score ranging from 0 to 100, with higher scores indicating more sleep problems [37].

To score the SPI II, you must first transform the responses of each item into a new score. For item 1, responses of 1, 2, 3, 4, and 5 are scored as 0, 25, 50, 75, and 100, respectively. For items 3 and 9, ratings of 1 through 6 are scored as 0, 20, 40, 60, 80, and 100, respectively. All of the other items are reverse-scored (lower ratings indicate more sleep difficulties) and so ratings of 1 through 6 for these items are scored as 100, 80, 60, 40, 20, and 0, respectively. The final SPI II score is an average of the item scores responded to.

Although the SPI II score can range from 0 to 100, the SPI II score is not a T-score (unlike the PROMIS measures, see Chapters 5 and 9). The mean of the SPI II score found in a nationally representative sample of 1011 US adults was 25.8 [38]. Research shows that, as would be expected, patients with chronic pain have higher mean SPI II scores, with one sample of patients with painful diabetic neuropathy having an average SPI II score of 48.8 [39] and two samples of patients with fibromyalgia – a pain condition with sleep problems as a central issue – having SPI II mean scores of 58.3 and 65.0 [40]. The standard deviation of the SPI II score is approximately 20 [36,39]. Thus, scores of 50–60 would indicate fairly significant sleep problems (1.0 and 1.5 standard deviation units higher than the normative sample), and changes of 10 or more (about 0.5 standard deviation units) would indicate meaningful change. A reasonable treatment goal, for patients reporting significant sleep problems, would be to reduce the SPI II score by at least 10 points, with an ultimate goal of having the final score be as close to 0 as possible, but at least below 30.

Medical Outcomes Study Sleep Problem Index II

	0–15 mins	16–30 mins	31–45 mins	46–60 mins	More than 60 mins	
1. How long did it usually take for you to fall asleep during the past 4 weeks?	1	2	3	4	5	
How often during the past 4 weeks did you… (circle one number on each line)	All of the time	Most of the time	A good portion of the time	Some of the time	A little of the time	None of the time
2. …feel that your sleep was not quiet (moving restlessly, feeling tense, speaking, etc., while sleeping)?	1	2	3	4	5	6
3. …get enough sleep to feel rested upon waking in the morning?	1	2	3	4	5	6
4. …awaken short of breath or with a headache?	1	2	3	4	5	6
5. …feel drowsy or sleepy during the day?	1	2	3	4	5	6
6. …have trouble falling asleep?	1	2	3	4	5	6
7. …awaken during your sleep time and have trouble falling asleep again?	1	2	3	4	5	6
8. …have trouble staying awake during the day?	1	2	3	4	5	6
9. …get the amount of sleep you needed?	1	2	3	4	5	6

Figure 7.1 **Medical Outcomes Study Sleep Problem Index II.** ©1986 RAND Corporation. Reproduced with permission from the RAND Corporation [37].

Chapter 8

Measuring depression

Estimates of patients with chronic pain who also have significant depression vary from 35% to 72%, depending on the sample and measure of depression used [41–43]. Although improvements in depression do not necessarily result in reductions in pain severity (in fact, the opposite pattern exists, with reductions in pain severity associated with subsequent reductions in depression [44]), treating depression can reduce the negative effects of pain on patient functioning [45]. Moreover, depression can contribute to the suffering associated with pain, and can interfere with motivation to engage in more active and adaptive pain coping responses [46,47]. When present, depression should be treated; and as indicated above, depression is present in many patients with chronic pain. A large number of measures of depression exist. One measure that is appropriate to use in a busy clinical setting is the Patient Health Questionnaire-2 (PHQ-2).

Patient Health Questionnaire-2

The original PHQ items were written to assess the presence and severity of each of the nine DSM-IV criteria for major depression, and it has demonstrated excellent accuracy (88%) for distinguishing patients with depression from those without depression [48]. Two of the PHQ Depression items (which make up the PHQ-2) have been shown to be almost as accurate [49], and represent a significant decrease in assessment burden over the 9-item PHQ Depression Scale; an issue of critical importance in many clinical situations. Moreover, the PHQ-2 has also demonstrated an ability to accurately reflect improvements and deterioration in depression outcomes and detect changes in depressive symptoms with treatment [50]. The PHQ-2 has also been validated in a sample of adolescents [51].

The two PHQ-2 items are presented on pain in Figure 8.1. The PHQ-2 score is simply the sum of each item's ratings, so that the score can range from 0 to 6. Using a cut-off point of 3 (i.e., scores of 2 or less indicating no depression and scores of 3 or more indicating the presence of depression), the PHQ-2 had demonstrated a sensitivity of 83% (among those with scores of 3 or higher, 83% meet criteria for major depression), and a specificity of 90% (among those with scores of 2 or less, 90% do not meet criteria for major depression) [49]. These accuracy rates compare favorably to the full 9-item PHQ Depression Scale as well as other measures of depression [52,53].

To help identify meaningful change scores in the PHQ-2, one study examined changes in depression diagnostic criteria in a sample of medical outpatients over a 1-year period, categorizing the patients as improved, unchanged, or deteriorated. Patients classified as "improved" over the 1-year period reported an average decrease of 2.3 on their PHQ-2 0–6 score. "Unchanged" participants reported an average decrease of 0.4, and "deteriorated" participants reported an average increase of 1.3. Thus, differences as low as 1 on the 0–6 score might be meaningful for some patients, and differences of about 2 are very likely meaningful.

Patient Health Questionnaire-2

Over the past two weeks, how often have you been bothered by the following problems?	Not at all	Several days	More than half the days	Nearly every day
1. Little interest or pleasure in doing things	0	1	2	3
2. Feeling down, depressed, or hopeless	0	1	2	3

Figure 8.1 Patient Health Questionnaire-2. Reproduced with permission from Kroenke et al. [49].

Chapter 9

Measuring general physical functioning

Physical functioning reflects the functioning of specific body parts (e.g., arms and hands, legs) as well as general ability to engage in instrumental activities such as cooking, cleaning, and running errands. Clinicians should consider assessing and monitoring global physical functioning in patients with pain problems for a number of reasons. First, physical functioning is influenced by pain, so improvements in physical functioning with pain treatment could be used as evidence for positive treatment outcome. At the same time, if substantial improvements in some pain domains – such as pain intensity – are observed, while little improvement in physical functioning is seen, this may be used as evidence that treatment may not be adequately broad enough to influence global rehabilitation.

A large number of measures of physical functioning exist. The 4- and 8-item PROMIS Short Form Physical Function scales are relatively recent additions to these measures. However, due to their careful construction as well as their flexibility and ease of interpretation, they are an excellent choice for many clinical settings.

PROMIS Physical Function Short Forms

The 4-item PROMIS Physical Function Short Form includes a list of four different physical functioning tasks (Figure 9.1). Patients respond to these items to indicate how much difficulty they had performing the task in the past week on a 5-point scale from "Without any difficulty" to "Unable to do." Each response has a score associated with it from 5 through 1 ("Without any difficulty" = 5; "With a little difficulty" = 4; "With some difficulty" = 3; "With much difficulty" = 2; "Unable to do" = 1).

The patient's raw physical functioning score is the sum of all items. Thus, the 4-item Short Form raw score can range from 4 to 20.

The 8-item PROMIS Physical Function Short Form (Figure 9.2) includes the items from the 4-item short form, as well as four additional items that ask patients to rate how much their physical health limits their ability to perform four activities on a 5-point scale ranging from "Not at all" to "Cannot do." Each response is scored from 5 through 1 ("Not at all" = 5; "Very little" = 4; "Somewhat" = 3; "Quite a bit" = 2; "Cannot do" = 1). The raw score sum of all eight items can range from 8 to 40.

Although both of the scales show excellent reliability and validity, a scale with more items has more overall precision. Thus, the 4-item Short Form may be most useful for screening or when assessment burden is a significant issue. The 8-item version may be more useful when assessment burden is less of an issue, or if an ability to detect smaller changes in physical functioning over time is critical. Tables 9.1 and 9.2 can be used to convert a patient's raw physical functioning score into T-scores for the 4- and 8-item versions, respectively. Note that the conversion table can only be used when a respondent completes all of the items in a scale.

The ideal endpoint goal for patients with chronic pain is to be able to function well (without difficulty or with little difficulty, and with no limits or very few limits on function) despite pain. This would translate to raw scores of 16 or higher (T-score 41.8 or higher) for the 4-item Physical Function scale and 32 (T-score 43.1 or higher) for the 8-item Physical Function scale. These would therefore be ideal endpoint goals, with increases in at least 5 T-score points (0.5 standard deviation units) representing meaningful improvements in physical function.

PROMIS Physical Function 4-item Short Form

Respond to each question by marking one box per row

	Without any difficulty	With a little difficulty	With some difficulty	With much difficulty	Unable to do
1. Are you able to do chores such as vacuuming or yard work?					
2. Are you able to go up and down stairs at a normal pace?					
3. Are you able to go for a walk of at least 15 minutes?					
4. Are you able to run errands and shop?					

Figure 9.1 PROMIS Physical Function 4-item Short Form. ©2009 PROMIS Health Organization and PROMIS Cooperative Group. Reproduced with permission from PROMIS [19].

PROMIS Physical Functioning 4-item Short Form conversion table

Raw score	T-score	SE
4	22.9	3.9
5	26.9	2.7
6	29.1	2.4
7	30.7	2.2
8	32.1	2.2
9	33.3	2.1
10	34.4	2.1
11	35.6	2.1
12	36.7	2.1
13	37.9	2.2
14	39.1	2.2
15	40.4	2.2
16	41.8	2.3
17	43.4	2.4
18	45.3	2.6
19	48.0	3.1
20	56.9	6.7

Table 9.1 PROMIS Physical Functioning 4-item Short Form conversion table. SE, standard error. ©2009 PROMIS Health Organization and PROMIS Cooperative Group. Reproduction with permission from PROMIS [19].

PROMIS Physical Function 8-item Short Form

Respond to each question by marking one box per row

	Without any difficulty	With a little difficulty	With some difficulty	With much difficulty	Unable to do
1. Are you able to do chores such as vacuuming or yard work?					
2. Are you able to go up and down stairs at a normal pace?					
3. Are you able to go for a walk of at least 15 minutes?					
4. Are you able to run errands and shop?					
	Not at all	Very little	Somewhat	Quite a lot	Cannot do
5. How much do physical health problems now limit your usual physical activities (such as walking or climbing stairs?					
6. Does your health now limit you in doing moderate work around the house like vacuuming, sweeping floors or carrying in groceries?					
7. Does your health now limit you in lifting or carrying groceries?					
8. Does your health now limit you in doing heavy work around the house like scrubbing floors, or lifting or moving heavy furniture?					

Figure 9.1 PROMIS Physical Function 8-item Short Form. ©2009 PROMIS Health Organization and PROMIS Cooperative Group. Reproduced with permission from PROMIS [19].

PROMIS Physical Functioning 8-item Short Form conversion table

Raw score	T-score	SE
8	20.2	3.5
9	23.7	2.4
10	25.6	2.1
11	27.0	1.9
12	28.2	1.8
13	29.3	1.8
14	30.3	1.7
15	31.2	1.7
16	32.0	1.6
17	32.7	1.6
18	33.5	1.6
19	34.2	1.6
20	34.9	1.6
21	35.5	1.5
22	36.2	1.5
23	36.9	1.5
24	37.5	1.5
25	38.2	1.5
26	38.9	1.5
27	39.5	1.5
28	40.2	1.6
29	40.9	1.6
30	41.6	1.6
31	42.4	1.6
32	43.1	1.6
33	43.9	1.6
34	44.8	1.7
35	45.7	1.8
36	46.8	1.9
37	48.0	2.1
38	49.6	2.5
39	51.8	2.9
40	59.2	6.1

Table 9.2 PROMIS Physical Functioning 8-item Short Form conversion table (continued).
SE, Standard error. ©2009 PROMIS Health Organization and PROMIS Cooperative Group.
Reproduced with permission from PROMIS [19].

Chapter 10

Measuring alcohol and drug use

A subset of patients with chronic pain use alcohol and other non-prescription drugs to cope with pain, and it is worthwhile to screen for this use when evaluating these patients. Two questions have demonstrated validity for this purpose, and an additional four questions can be asked to help evaluate the extent of alcohol use, if indicated.

Two-item conjoint screen

A two-item conjoint screen (TICS) for alcohol and other drug problems consists of the two questions presented in Figure 10.1 [54]. Scoring is easy; you simply sum the number of affirmative responses to these questions; the score can therefore range from 0 to 2. In the scale development sample, scores of 0, 1, and 2 were associated with a 7.3%, 36.5%, and 72.4% chance, respectively, of having a current substance abuse disorder [54]. A version of TICS that asks only about alcohol use has demonstrated validity via strong associations with serious alcohol-related behaviors in a large sample of veterans [55]. Positive responses to either or both questions can be followed up with additional questions to determine the extent of alcohol or drug use.

Behavioral Risk Factor Surveillance System assessing alcohol use

The Centers for Disease Control and Prevention (CDC) performs an annual survey of health risk factors, called the Behavioral Risk Factor Surveillance System survey (www.cdc.gov/brfss/questionnaires). Four of these questions ask about alcohol use and are presented in Figure 10.2.

The first question is a general screening question, and might be skipped if you already know that the patient drank at least one alcoholic beverage in the past 30 days (note, in 2009, 54.4% of a representative sample indicated that they drank one alcoholic beverage in the past 30 days). The second question allows you to determine overall frequency of drinking. Questions 3 and 4 can be used to classify patients as a "heavy" drinker or a "binge" drinker. Classification as either suggests the need for a reduction in alcohol use, perhaps facilitated by alcohol treatment. Adult men who have three or more drinks per day (on the days that they drink) and adult women who have two or more drinks per day (on the days that they drink) meet criteria for being heavy drinkers (nationwide in 2009, 5.1% of a national representative sample of men and of women met criteria for being heavy drinkers). A "binge" drinker is someone who responds with a number greater than 0 to question 4 (nationwide in 2009, 15.8% in a national representative sample met criteria for being binge drinkers).

Two-item conjoint screen for assessing alcohol and drug use

- In the last year, have you ever drunk or used drugs more than you meant to?
- Have you felt you wanted or needed to cut down on your drinking or drug use in the last year?

Figure 10.1 Two-item conjoint screen for assessing alcohol and drug use.

CDC Behavioral Risk Factor Surveillance System assessing alcohol use

1. During the past 30 days, have you had at least one drink of any alcoholic beverage such as beer, wine, a malt beverage, or liquor?

2. During the past 30 days, how many days per week or per month did you have at least one drink of any alcoholic beverage?

3. One drink is equivalent to a 12-ounce beer, a 5-ounce glass of wine, or a drink with one shot of liquor. During the past 30 days, on the days when you drank, about how many drinks did you drink on the average? **(Note: A 40-ounce beer would count as 3 drinks, or a cocktail drink with 2 shots would count as 2 drinks.)**

4. Considering all types of alcoholic beverages, how many times during the past 30 days did you have **X (X = 5 for men, X = 4 for women)** or more drinks on one occasion?

Metric conversion: 12 ounce = 355 mL

Figure 10.2 CDC Behavioral Risk Factor Surveillance System assessing alcohol use.

Measuring global improvement and satisfaction with pain care

All of the measures described up to this point assess a specific domain that clinicians should consider measuring and monitoring in their patients with pain. None provide a general global assessment of how the patient views his or her overall pain management program, or the most recent pain treatment he or she received. The assessment of global improvement and satisfaction with treatment is now considered important in pain clinical trials, in part because this allows patients to communicate overall satisfaction with care, taking into account not only treatment-related improvements in pain, but also other factors, such as the presence and severity of side effects, as well as the relationship with the care providers [56,57]. Clinicians may also determine that a global assessment of satisfaction with pain care is useful for monitoring ongoing treatment efficacy.

Five-point patient rating of satisfaction with pain management

A 5-point verbal patient rating scale of satisfaction with their general pain management and the same scale assessing satisfaction with a specific treatment are presented in Figures 11.1 and 11.2, respectively. When using these scales, patients are asked to indicate the word or phrase that best describes their overall satisfaction with their pain management program or their most recent pain treatment, respectively. Responses can be then coded from 0 to 4, where 0 = "Very dissatisfied," 1 = "Dissatisfied," 2 = "Neutral," 3 = "Satisfied," and 4 = "Very satisfied." Any ratings indicating a lack of satisfaction (e.g., 0 or 1) can then be followed up to determine if changes in treatment or changes in treatment goals (i.e., more realistic) are indicated.

Patient Global Impression of Change

One of the most common measures of patient global impression of change is the Patient Global Impression of Change scale (Figure 11.3). Using this scale, the patient can indicate whether, and the extent to which, there has been a change in pain for the worse or better since the last visit (or in the last month, week, or day, etc.). To administer the scale, you simply ask the patient, *"How would you rate the change in your pain in the last _____ day(s)/week(s)/month(s)/since your last visit?"*, and ask the patient to indicate this on a 7-point verbal rating scale from "much worse" to "much better." Interpretation of the responses to the scale are clear. Ratings showing a perceived worsening in the pain problem, especially in light of significant increases in pain intensity (see Chapter 2) or any one of the other outcome domain measures described in this handbook, require a more in-depth evaluation to determine the reason(s) for this worsening, and these reasons should be addressed, where possible.

Patient rating of satisfaction with pain management

How would you rate your overall satisfaction with your pain management program?

☐ Very dissatisfied

☐ Dissatisfied

☐ Neutral

☐ Satisfied

☐ Very satisfied

Figure 11.1 Patient rating of satisfaction with pain management.

Patient rating of satisfaction with a specific pain treatment

How would you rate your overall satisfaction with the most recent pain treatment you received?

☐ Very dissatisfied

☐ Dissatisfied

☐ Neutral

☐ Satisfied

☐ Very satisfied

Figure 11.2 Patient rating of satisfaction with a specific pain treatment.

Patient Global Impression of Change scale

How would you rate the change in your pain in the last _____ day(s)/week(s)/month(s)/ since your last visit?

☐ Much worse

☐ Worse

☐ A little worse

☐ No change

☐ A little better

☐ Better

☐ Much better

Figure 11.3 Patient Global Impression of Change scale.

References

1 Phillips C, Main C, Buck R, et al. Prioritising pain in policy making: the need for a whole systems perspective. *Health Policy* 2008;88:166–75.

2 Stewart WF, Ricci JA, Chee E, et al. Lost productive time and cost due to common pain conditions in the US workforce. *JAMA* 2003;290:2443–54.

3 Lippe PM, Brock C, David J, et al. The First National Pain Medicine Summit-final summary report. *Pain Medicine* 2010;11:1447–68.

4 Jensen MP. Pain assessment in clinical trials. In: *Pain Management: Evidence, Outcomes, and Quality of Life in Pain Treatment*. Edited by H Wittink and D Carr. Amsterdam: Elsevier, 2008;57–88.

5 Jensen MP. Measurement of pain. In: *Bonica's management of pain*. Edited by SM Fishman, et al. Philadelphia, PA: Williams & Wilkins Media, 2010;251–70.

6 de C Williams AC, Davies HT, Chadury Y. Simple pain rating scales hide complex idiosyncratic meanings. *Pain* 2000;85:457–63.

7 Serlin RC, Mendoza TR, Nakamura Y, et al. When is cancer pain mild, moderate or severe? Grading pain severity by its interference with function. *Pain* 1995;61:277–84.

8 Farrar JT, Portenoy RK, Berlin JA, et al. Defining the clinically important difference in pain outcome measures. *Pain* 2000;88:287–94.

9 Hicks CL, von Baeyer CL, Spafford P, et al. The FACES Pain Scale - Revised: Toward a common metric in pediatric pain measurement. *Pain* 2001;93:173–83.

10 Dworkin RH, O'Connor AB, Audette J, et al. Recommendations for the pharmacological management of neuropathic pain: an overview and literature update. *Mayo Clin Proc* 2010;85:S3–14.

11 Chou R. Pharmacological management of low back pain. *Drugs* 2010;70:387–402.

12 Jensen MP, Galer B, Gammaitoni A. *The Pain Quality Assessment Scale (PQAS) and Revised Pain Quality Assessment Scale (PQAS-R): Manual and User Guide 2010*. Available at www.mapi-trust. org/services/questionnairelicensing/cataloguequestionnaires/150-pqasr. [Last accessed 15th April 2011]

13 Bennett M. The LANSS Pain Scale: the Leeds Assessment of Neuropathic Symptoms and Signs. *Pain* 2001;92:147–57.

14 Potter J, Higginson IJ, Scadding JW, et al. Identifying neuropathic pain in patients with head and neck cancer: use of the Leeds Assessment of Neuropathic Symptoms and Signs Scale. *J R Soc Med* 2003;96:379–83.

15 Yucel A, Senocak M, Kocasoy Orhan E, et al. Results of the Leeds assessment of neuropathic symptoms and signs pain scale in Turkey: a validation study. *J Pain* 2004;5:427–32.

16 Toomey TC, Gover VF, Jones BN. Spatial distribution of pain: a descriptive characteristic of chronic pain. *Pain* 1983;17:289–300.

17 Revicki DA, Chen WH, Harnam N, et al. Development and psychometric analysis of the PROMIS pain behavior item bank. *Pain* 2009;146:158–69.

18 Dworkin RH, Turk DC, Wynwich KW, et al. Interpreting the clinical importance of treatment outcomes in chronic pain clinical trials: IMMPACT recommendations. *J Pain* 2008;9:105–21.

19 PROMIS Health Organization and PROMIS Cooperative Group. *PROMIS Scoring Manuals.* Available at www.assessmentcenter.net/Manuals.aspx. [Last accessed 15th April 2011]

20 Cleeland CS. *The Brief Pain Inventory User Guide 2009.* Available at www.mdanderson.org/education-and-research/departments-programs-and-labs/departments-and-divisions/symptom-research/symptom-assessment-tools/BPI_UserGuide.pdf [Last accessed 15th April 2011]

21 Tyler EJ, Jensen MP, Engel JM, et al. The reliability and validity of pain interference measures in persons with cerebral palsy. *Arch Phys Med Rehabil* 2002;83:236–9.

22 Hanley MA, Masedo A, Jensen MP, et al. Pain interference in persons with spinal cord injury: Classification of mild, moderate, and severe pain. *J Pain* 2006;7:129–33.

23 Raichle K, Osborne TL, Jensen MP, et al. The reliability and validity of pain interference measures in persons with spinal cord injury. *J Pain* 2006;7:179–86.

24 World Health Organization. *International Classification of Functioning, Disability and Health (ICF).* Geneva: World Health Organization. 2008;iii:299. Available at www.who.int/classifications/icf/en/. [Last accessed 15th April 2011]

25 Osborne TL, Raichle KA, Jensen MP, et al. The reliability and validity of pain interference measures in persons with multiple sclerosis. *J Pain Symptom Manage* 2006;32:217–29.

26 Lim JY, Tchai E, Jang SN. Effectiveness of aquatic exercise for obese patients with knee osteoarthritis: a randomized controlled trial. *PM&R* 2010;2:723–31 (quiz 793).

27 Lin HY, Cheng TT, Wang JH, et al. Etoricoxib improves pain, function and quality of life: results of a real-world effectiveness trial. *Int J Rheum Dis* 2010;13:144–50.

28 Arnold LM, Goldenberg DL, Stanford SB, et al. Gabapentin in the treatment of fibromyalgia: a randomized, double-blind, placebo-controlled, multicenter trial. *Arthritis Rheum* 2007;56:1336–44.

29 Breivik H, Collett B, Ventafridda V, et al. Survey of chronic pain in Europe: prevalence, impact on daily life, and treatment. *Eur J Pain* 2006;10:287–333.

30 Atkinson JH, Ancoli-Israel S, Slater MA, et al. Subjective sleep disturbance in chronic back pain. *Clin J Pain* 1988;65:225–32.

31 Smith MT, Perlis ML, Smith MS, et al. Sleep quality and presleep arousal in chronic pain. *J Behav Med* 2000;23:1–13.

32 Lunde LH, Pallesen S, Krangnes L, et al. Characteristics of sleep in older persons with chronic pain: a study based on actigraphy and self-reporting. *Clin J Pain* 2010;26:132–7.

33 O'Brien EM, Waxenberg LB, Atchison JW, et al. Negative mood mediates the effect of poor sleep on pain among chronic pain patients. *Clin J Pain* 2010;26:310–9.

34 Onen SH, Onen F, Albrand G, et al. Pain tolerance and obstructive sleep apnea in the elderly. *J Am Med Dir Assoc* 2010;11:612–6.

35 Vitiello MV, Rybarczyk B, Von Korff M, et al. Cognitive behavioral therapy for insomnia improves sleep and decreases pain in older adults with co-morbid insomnia and osteoarthritis. *J Clin Sleep Med* 2009;5:355–62.

36 Hays RD, Stewart AL (Editors). Sleep measures. In: *Measuring Functioning and Well-Being: The Medical Outcomes Study Approach.* Durham, NC: Duke University Press, 1992;235–59.

37 Spritzer KL, Hays RD. *MOS Sleep Scale: A Manual for Use and Scoring, Version 1.0.* Los Angeles, CA: RAND, 2003.

38 Hays RD, Martin S, Sesti SA, et al. Psychometric properties of the Medical Outcomes Study Sleep measure. *Sleep Med* 2005;6:41–4.

39 Viala-Danten M, Martin S, Guillemin I, et al. Evaluation of the reliability and validity of the Medical Outcomes Study sleep scale in patients with painful diabetic peripheral neuropathy during an international clinical trial. *Health Qual Life Outcomes* 2008;6:113.

40 Russell IJ, Crofford LJ, Leon T, et al. The effects of pregabalin on sleep disturbance symptoms among individuals with fibromyalgia syndrome. *Sleep Med* 2009;10:604–10.

41 Castro M, Kraychete D, Daltro C, et al. Comorbid anxiety and depression disorders in patients with chronic pain. *Arq Neuropsiquiatr* 2009;67:982–5.

42 Miller LR, Cano A. Comorbid chronic pain and depression: who is at risk? *J Pain* 2009;10:619–27.
43 Poole H, White S, Blake C, et al. Depression in chronic pain patients: prevalence and measurement. *Pain Pract* 2009;9:173–80.
44 Fishbain DA, Cutler R, Rosomoff HL, et al. Chronic pain-associated depression: antecedent or consequence of chronic pain? A review. *Clin J Pain* 1997;13:116–37.
45 Teh CF, Zaslavsky AM, Reynolds CF, et al. Effect of depression treatment on chronic pain outcomes. *Psychosom Med* 2010;72:61–7.
46 Bair MJ, Matthias MS, Nyland KA, et al. Barriers and facilitators to chronic pain self-management: a qualitative study of primary care patients with comorbid musculoskeletal pain and depression. *Pain Medicine* 2009;10:1280–90.
47 Tennen H, Affleck G, Zautra A. Depression history and coping with chronic pain: a daily process analysis. *Health Psychology* 2006;25:370–9.
48 Kroenke K, Spitzer RL, Williams JB. The PHQ-9: validity of a brief depression severity measure. *J Gen Intern Med* 2001;16:606–13.
49 Kroenke K, Spitzer RL, Williams JB. The Patient Health Questionnaire-2: validity of a two-item depression screener. *Med Care* 2003;41:1284–92.
50 Lowe B, Kroenke K, Grafe K. Detecting and monitoring depression with a two-item questionnaire (PHQ-2). *J Psychoso Res* 2005;58:163–71.
51 Richardson LP, Rockhill C, Russo JE, et al. Evaluation of the PHQ-2 as a brief screen for detecting major depression among adolescents. *Pediatrics* 2010;125:e1097–103.
52 Boyle LL, Richardson TM, He H, et al. How do the PHQ-2, the PHQ-9 perform in aging services clients with cognitive impairment? *Int J Geriatr Psychiatry* 2010;[epub].
53 Smith MV, Gotman N, Lin H, et al. Do the PHQ-8 and the PHQ-2 accurately screen for depressive disorders in a sample of pregnant women? *Gen Hosp Psych* 2010;32:544–8.
54 Brown RL, Leonard T, Saunders LA, et al. A two-item conjoint screen for alcohol and other drug problems. *J Am Board Fam Pract* 2001;14:95–106.
55 Santiago PN, Wilk JE, Milliken CS, et al., Screening for alcohol misuse and alcohol-related behaviors among combat veterans. *Psychiatr Serv* 2010;61:575–81.
56 Turk DC, Dworkin RH, Allen RR, et al. Core outcome domains for chronic pain clinical trials: IMMPACT recommendations. *Pain* 2003;106:337–45.
57 Dworkin RH, Turk DC, Farrar JT, et al. Core outcome measures for chronic pain clinical trials: IMMPACT recommendations. *Pain* 2005;113:9–19.